Ministerial round table on diet, physical activity and health,

Regional Commitee for the Western Pacific
Fifty-third Session
Kyoto, Japan, 16-20 September 2002

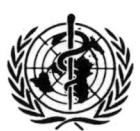

World Health Organization
Regional Office for the Western Pacific
2003

WHO Library Cataloguing in Publication Data

Ministerial round table on diet, physical activity and health,
Regional Commitee for the Western Pacific, 53rd session,
16-20 September 2002

1. Chronic disease -- prevention and control 2. Diet 3. Exercise
4. Life style

ISBN 92 9061 046 8   (NLM Classification: WT 500)

© World Health Organization 2003

All rights reserved.

The designations employed and the presentation of the material in this publication do not imply the expression of any opinion whatsoever on the part of the World Health Organization concerning the legal status of any country, territory, city or area or of its authorities, or concerning the delimitation of its frontiers or boundaries.

The mention of specific companies or of certain manufacturers' products does not imply that they are endorsed or recommended by the World Health Organization in preference to others of a similar nature that are not mentioned. Errors and omissions excepted, the names of proprietary products are distinguished by initial capital letters.

The World Health Organization does not warrant that the information contained in this publication is complete and correct and shall not be liable for any damages incurred as a result of its use.

Publications of the World Health Organization can be obtained from Marketing and Dissemination, World Health Organization, 20 Avenue Appia, 1211 Geneva 27, Switzerland (tel: +41 22 791 2476; fax: +41 22 791 4857; email: bookorders@who.int). Requests for permission to reproduce WHO publications, in part or in whole, or to translate them – whether for sale or for noncommercial distribution – should be addressed to Publications, at the above address (fax: +41 22 791 4806; email: permissions@who.int).

CONTENTS

Introduction	5
A strategy for the prevention and control of noncommunicable diseases: A new challenge	7
Physical activity and exercise: The enabling instruments	13
Narrative summary of comments by representatives	18
Barriers and actions needed to improve health status through diet and physical activity	23
Summary of other comments	28
Recommendation to WHO	29

(blank page)

INTRODUCTION

In countries of the Western Pacific Region, undernutrition and micronutrient deficiencies are still important components of the burden of disease, especially for young children. However, in most countries, the chronic diseases of adulthood already constitute the main burden for health and health services. Diet and physical activity are two key factors contributing to this disease burden.

At the fifty-third session of the Regional Committee for the Western Pacific in Kyoto, Japan, health policy-makers from 30 countries and areas of the Western Pacific participated in a round table on "Diet, Physical Activity and Health". The round table discussed how lifestyle changes can be achieved in whole populations. Reviewing successful experiences, participants stressed the need to build supportive environments to facilitate personal change. Many factors generate changes in disease patterns; to bring about positive changes in lifestyles it will take an alliance of many partners, in government, the private sector and civil society.

This summary of ideas and experiences discussed at the Ministerial Round table will be one of the contributions from the Western Pacific Region to developing a global strategy on diet, physical activity and health.

Shigeru Omi, MD, Ph.D.
Regional Director
WHO Regional Office
for the Western Pacific

(blank page)

A STRATEGY FOR THE PREVENTION AND CONTROL OF NONCOMMUNICABLE DISEASES: A NEW CHALLENGE

Dr W. Philip T. James
Director, Public Health Policy Group/
Chairman, International Obesity Task Force, England

The Asian challenge

The escalating chronic diseases of adulthood are now the principal health burdens in the Asia-Pacific region. They already dominate health services and will increase markedly over the next 20 years. Governments should regard their populations as unusually prone to excessive weight gain and particularly abdominal obesity, type 2 diabetes, hypertension, ischaemic heart disease and strokes. There is reasonably clear evidence that these diseases are more severe and appear earlier in Asia than in other regions; probably because of the unusual combination of intergenerational mild to severe malnutrition of women and their children in combination with the sudden transition in eating habits and activity patterns. The health burdens caused by these diseases are probably increasing more rapidly in Asia than anywhere else in the world and governments can no longer ignore the problem. The question is: what should they be doing?

The dilemmas facing prevention

There are three dilemmas: first, the assumption that prevention is slow and its effects small. This is wrong. Second, it is not often understood that the greatest health gains for a country usually come from changing the behaviour of the average family, rather than from focusing on high-risk groups. Third, the causes of the Asian epidemic of chronic diseases are environmental, so they need to be remedied by extensive measures, including some taken by ministries outside the health sector. Health services often have to cope with the consequences of other government policies.

The causes of noncommunicable diseases: the pressures

Foods and drinks have an increasing energy density. This is because of reductions in the intake of vegetables, fruit and other high-fibre starchy foods and increases in animal fats, vegetable oils and sugars or syrups in poorer quality foods and drinks. Intensive marketing and changing cultural perceptions are contributing to the retreat from Asian foods. Physical activity is falling rapidly because of the systematic and highly successful measures by governments and commerce to reduce the need for physical work in the home, in transport and at the workplace. The challenge for ministries of health therefore is to work out the principal forces and processes involved and, where possible, to develop, with other ministries, measures which include effective public/private partnerships. These should include methods of handling any industrial group which does not adapt its products and approaches and uses techniques to confuse, question or obstruct change. The health costs of chronic diseases are now the concern of ministries of finance, but many do not have access to health impact assessments of different options for change. Nor have many ministries of health managed to nurture the public, the media or the politically-active sector to gain the backing needed for change.

A new approach: define the principal drivers of both sedentary behaviour and the passive over consumption of energy-dense diets

To consider where changes are needed, first the principal contributors to fat, saturated fat, salt and syrup sugar intakes need to be assessed. This then allows targeting of (1) appropriate food and drink, and (2) the locations where these are consumed, e.g. home, school, work or "fast food" outlets. Table 1 provides a format for considering the major issues relating to physical facilities and the arrangements for food provision and physical activity. It includes economic issues requiring the ministry of health or associated ministries to contribute public funds or to specify charging schemes for public services. Policy development and socio-cultural issues are treated as separate categories. Socio-cultural issues are included because policy-makers are often concerned that particular sectors of society may have an inappropriate perception or a culturally-based conviction that a particular approach to a problem is appropriate or wrong. In such cases, health education, advocacy and promotional campaigns can be useful. Table 1 therefore simply illustrates the way that a ministry of health can think through the problems of how best to deal with critical issues requiring change; recognizing that some can be dealt with by altering funding priorities within the ministry, adopting new regulatory arrangements or by providing public information in an innovative way. Others are the responsibility of other ministers; the evidence from recent food safety problems shows the need for civil society backing for ministries of health when negotiating with other powerful ministries.

Major issues to be considered in relation to food and drink

Major issues to be considered in relation to food and drink include:

- Nutritional management of disease: criteria and drug use; health of medical personnel

- Facilities and standards of education and food provision for schoolchildren

- Breast-feeding promotion and controls on marketing to pre-school children

- Novel approaches to public and private sector catering; controls on restaurants

- Fast foods and drinks; safety, control options; pricing policies
- The rural/urban transition and its effects on food availability; strategies for change
- Local food production and food manufacturing for health
- Urban planning as towns and cities grow rapidly: avoiding "food deserts" for the poor.
- Simple food labelling and standards; role of the Ministry of Health in the Codex Alimentarius Commission and the World Trade Organization
- Physical issues to be considered in avoiding sedentary states
- Physical issues to be considered in relation to avoiding sedentary states include:
- Prescribing exercise for staff and patients: promoting new evidence of benefits of exercise
- Hospital and health centre facilities in Asia: facilitating cycling and public transport
- Public and private sector workers' facilities: facilitating routine exercise
- School environments, facilities, priorities in education; considering sex differences
- Transport policies: making streets safe, controlling car use, promoting walking and cycling
- Work-based initiatives and transport to work

Taking the initiative and ensuring progress

Many health initiatives fail because governments develop them in response to new demands for action. However, new priorities soon divert the attention of ministers and senior officials. In practice progress is rarely made without involving the "four Ps": politicians, professionals, press and public. International experience, for example in Thailand in combating childhood malnutrition, shows that dramatic progress can be made if there is wide media, local government and community involvement. For example, ministries of health may chose to recruit an independent activist group or institution of professionals with civil society involvement to maintain momentum and provide ministries of health with political support. This is particularly important if health ministries are to gain effective cooperation from other ministries, for example education, agriculture, trade, transport, economic development or finance, where health priorities are rarely considered and where the responses to health proposals on chronic diseases are often seen in terms of the need for "health education". There is a need to redefine health impact assessments, taking into account other government departments' policies, and to change the perception of the health sector as a cost to government to a societal investment. Thus health issues are often seen by governments as being less significant than an offer of investment or trade opportunities in agriculture, food manufacturing or retailing. Both affluent and less affluent countries in the Region are faced with alarming projections for disease and disability which could be combated by retaining many features of traditional Asian diets and not following the disastrous policies of Western countries.

Table 1

	Ministry of Health's direct responsibilities			Other ministries: specified on a national basis		
	Dietary quality; physical activity	Food safety/nutrition	Environmental health issues	Physical activity; Dietary quality;	Food safety/ nutrition	Environmental health issues
Physical	Appropriately accessible health centres Promoting access to appropriate self-monitoring systems e.g. weight, blood pressure	Catering in hospitals; monitoring facilities	Fluoridation systems for water Facilities for iodizing salt	Ensuring playgrounds in schools, suitable cycling and road systems; urban planning; sports facilities Designated urban areas for local food production	Provision of appropriate local abattoirs Proper public toilet and sanitary facilities Proper catering facilities based on stringent hygiene requirements. Link to nutritional needs	Urban planning: green spaces, cycle paths, parks, playgrounds, lead-free air Establish facilities for farmers' markets
Economic	Primary health payments for specific targets in management	Penalties for providing unsafe food; sales and tax policies in relation to nutritional quality of different food groups	Subsidize iodine for iodination purposes	Re-evaluate taxation and subsidy policies	Establish appropriate penalties for inappropriate hygiene	Consider agricultural subsidies/ taxes in health terms Finance new public transport systems Promote urban agriculture, new outlets for high quality, affordable foods in deprived areas
Policy	Baby-friendly Hospitals Dietary guidelines Establishing fortification policies Establish policies on health claims, e.g. functional foods	Health impact of multisectoral food safety policies	Establish specific guidelines for toxicants and contaminants in soil water and primary food products Health impact assessment of agrochemical use	Health impact assessments of agricultural developments Food labeling with appropriate, understandable health-related information	Establish criteria for ensuring pathogen and contaminant-free access to the food chain Establish systematic hazard analysis critical control point (HACCP) for food chain, systematic surveillance and mechanisms for emergency response	Reform agriculture policies Develop soil improvement, clean water, agricultural recycling, planting, fertilizer, pesticide, water use policies
Socio-cultural	Health education	Promote concept of limited clinical antibiotic use	Promote new concept of health impact of new traffic policy	Promote physical activity in the workplace Create breastfeeding time and space in the workplace with NGO help	Establish new criteria for excluding antibiotics as growth promoters and specifying veterinary use Educational initiatives for safety of fast food outlets, modifying nutrient composition, and limiting and ensuring appropriate food waste disposal	Change attitudes to cycle path use, pedestrian areas Educational initiatives for caterers, communal use of school recreational facilities

PHYSICAL ACTIVITY AND EXERCISE—THE ENABLING INSTRUMENTS

Datuk Dr M Jegathesan
Chief Executive Officer, Sistem Hospital Awasan Taraf
(A Health Facilities Consulting Company), Malaysia
Adjunct Professor, Faculty of Medicine and Health Sciences,
University Putra Malaysia

Physical activity and exercise are recognized to be health-enhancing activities that promise not only to add 'years to one's life' but also 'life to one's years'. The principles governing their application have been evolving but are now fairly well understood. The global promotion of healthy lifestyles is making progress but has not yet reached all societies. There are barriers dividing knowledge and its application at both community and individual levels.

At the individual level, clearly there are many who do not have access to knowledge about healthy behaviour and hence are not in a position to adopt it. However, even those who know about healthy behaviour often show 'inertia', and a lack of motivation to practice it. We can call this the 'knowledge/behaviour paradox'.

At the community level, barriers to implementation include lack of political will, absence of conviction, opposing interests (both political and economic), inadequate resources, and inappropriate criteria for prioritizing resource allocation.

Strategies for individuals and communities

Health authorities have to find strategies that will be able to bridge these gaps. Health-enhancing activities, far from being difficult to implement, can be readily integrated into most people's lives by making relatively minor adjustments to daily routines. They need not necessarily be expensive in terms of time or money. On an individual level, all that is required is the personal decision to make the change, the commitment to see it through and the motivation to sustain it. While such personal involvement will benefit the individual, wide public health impact can only be achieved if healthy behaviour is practised by large sectors of the population. For this, the government and public authorities have to provide awareness, expertise and an enabling or facilitating environment.

What it takes

To enjoy the benefits of an exercise programme, all that needs to be done is for about 30 minutes, three to four times per week, to be allocated to appropriate exercise. This is the minimum requirement. Effective exercise does not have to be done in a single block of time and can be split into two or three ten-minute sessions per day. Nor does it always have to be formal, regulated activity. Much exercise can be done in an opportunistic way by, for example, walking instead of riding, taking the stairs instead of elevators, etc.

The role of health policy-makers

National policies

Although many of the ingredients needed for holistic implementation of healthy lifestyle programmes are the responsibility of various agencies and ministries, health policy-makers and managers can play an important catalytic role. They can have an effect across the entire spectrum, from national policies to influencing the behaviour of individuals.

Mechanisms for coordination

A mechanism needs be created for this multisectoral collaboration and cooperation. One example would be a national fitness council, which could cut across several ministries or agencies. The tenets healthy lifestyle concept will need to be integrated into existing national policies covering health, development, education, town planning, sports, housing, human resources, transport, etc. It can become part of existing programmes such as 'healthy cities' and 'healthy workplaces'.

Successful execution of this could be through a spectrum of interaction ranging from promotion (and advocacy), persuasion, pressure, to penalties (through legislation).

The enabling environment: facilities and programmes

The 'enabling environment' that needs be created will include the provision for facilities, equity of physical and economic access to them, and removal of obstacles for their use. Facilities would include recreational parks as well as mandatory facilities in housing areas, schools, universities and workplaces. Facility provision must go hand in hand with programmes that will facilitate and encourage their use. This will include introducing, reintroducting or re-emphasizing activities such as physical education in schools, competitive and recreational sports in institutions and exercise breaks in workplaces. Conditions should be in place to encourage the use of public transport, cycling and walking.

Motivation

Facilities and programmes will only have an impact if users are motivated. Hence awareness and promotional campaigns using the power of the media, the Internet and advertising are needed. So too are events encouraging mass participation especially involving entire families. Programmes and facilities will have to take into consideration cultural and social sensitivities. They can be augmented by incentives ranging from tax breaks for fitness-related expenses, discounts off insurance premiums for 'healthy behaviour', appropriate recognition and rewards such as inclusion in the criteria for university admissions and career promotions.

Strategic partnerships

Apart from intersectoral collaboration and coordination there is a need for strategic partnerships with the private sector and with NGOs. Movements promoting 'family values' and combating substance abuse can make powerful allies.

Sport/fitness axis

The relationship between national sporting prowess and fitness in the population at large needs to be examined. This should be synergistic, with each nourishing and feeding on each other. A generally fit nation should provide a broader base from which athletic excellence can emerge, while sports heroes should serve as examples and encourage the adoption of active lifestyles. That is, if love for sports is not confined to the couch in front of the TV.

Fitness culture

The end result should be the evolution of a 'fitness culture'. For this, a sustained and relentless effort will be needed. The use of role models such as sports personalities, senior athletes, elite disabled athletes and community and political leaders should be maximized.

Leadership by example

In this regard, health policy- and decision-makers will give their advocacy roles a great boost if they can be seen as 'living examples' of what they are advocating.

Conclusion

Embracing the route to a healthy lifestyle is one of the most important personal decisions that one can make. It is a practice that is eminently applicable. The inputs in time and effort that an individual needs to make are small compared to the tremendous benefits that can be achieved.

However, individuals need an environment that will empower, enable and facilitate and motivate them. This is the responsibility of the civil authorities. For the nation, modest investments in policies and programmes will bring great dividends in terms of increased health, well-being and productivity of the population at large.

NARRATIVE SUMMARY OF COMMENTS BY REPRESENTATIVES

The ministerial round table discussion on diet, physical activity and health was attended by representatives of all delegations attending the 53rd WHO Regional Committee Meeting held in Kyoto, Japan, in September 2002. Representatives of 19 delegations made statements.

There was a remarkable consensus among the representatives that the prevalence of obesity-related diseases such as cardiovascular diseases, diabetes mellitus and cancer correlates directly to poor nutrition and physical inactivity. Several Member States expressed further that unhealthy diet and physical inactivity pose risks throughout life, and recognized that poor nutrition in early life and in utero could increase the risk of chronic disease in adulthood.

On the dietary and nutrition aspect of obesity, the most common barrier identified by Member States against a balanced diet and healthful eating habits was the availability and introduction of "fatty" and "empty calorie" foods, such as those catered by Western-type fast-food chains, and certain agricultural, meat and dairy products, including processed foods.

The role played by the media was another barrier commonly addressed by the representatives, particularly its role in popularizing the patronage of fast food, cigarette smoking, alcohol consumption and fashionable body images.

Some representatives also noted that these dietary trends do not always result in obesity but can lead to inadequate nutritional intake, particularly among women and adolescents.

Poor public awareness about nutrition, in general, is aggravated further by the substantial disjunction in many countries between the recognition of these major dietary problems and the lack of will to implement substantial changes that would have a significant impact on public health, i.e. the 'knowledge-behaviour' paradox and the potential conflict with customs and traditions.

Lifestyle changes, e.g. from an agricultural setting to office environs, and the increasing employment rate among women, especially those of child-bearing age, affect the dietary patterns of entire populations throughout the life cycle. On the other hand, in many countries a sizeable proportion of the population continues to live in poverty, encumbered by prohibitive food costs.

On the aspect of living a lifestyle characterized by physical activity, modern-day barriers most commonly referred to by representatives were higher income and better standards of living that afford technological advancement in the form of labour-saving amenities and devices, e.g. vehicles, lifts and automated appliances. These, coupled with diminishing space and time for physical recreation and movement, e.g. parks, pedestrian lanes, public transport, etc, further aggravate the matter.

Several representatives reported that their countries are now confronted with the "double-burden" of disease. While communicable diseases have not been completely eradicated in many populations, the prevalence of noncommunicable diseases has reached alarming proportions, the treatment of which absorbs an increasing share of national health budgets. The asymptomatic nature of obesity-related diseases until its late stages further complicates matters.

Other noteworthy observations forwarded by the representatives were inadequate support for nutrition research, the lack of trained health professionals in nutrition and physical activity and the misconception that health is the concern of national health ministries alone.

In response, representatives broadly called for the integration of health promotion strategies into national policies involving the health, agriculture, development, education, housing, town planning, sports, human resources, transport and tourism sectors. It was proposed that health impact assessments should form part of the policy requirement for all major planning and development processes, in the same way as environmental impact assessments do, which are now in place in most nations. In relation, strategic partnerships should be steadily fostered among all levels of government, industry and the non-government sectors, including establishments that have a direct effect on the eating behaviour of children and young people, e.g. grocery organizations, school canteens and fast food outlets. Special attention was proposed for building alliances with appropriate segments of the food industry, as opposed to taking an adversarial approach.

In promoting health consciousness and awareness, there was broad consensus on the need for sustained creative and relevant communications strategies to penetrate primary settings such as the home, pre-schools, schools and workplaces. Other strategies include promoting food labeling; the provision of incentives and awards for effective programmes and initiatives; the popularization of traditional cooking techniques, healthy recipes, traditional dances and martial arts exercises; and the use of role models, e.g. government officials, national personalities and sports celebrities.

Specifically in the realm of physical activity, representatives called for investing in infrastructure development for the creation of environments that enable and promote movement. There should be creativity in organizing national fitness events such as walkathons and hiking expeditions. Linking with tobacco-free-sports, smoking bans may be expanded gradually to cover all public areas.

And in order to augment public funds for infrastructure development, commercial partnerships may yield financial sponsorships, while tax deductions for expenses in physical activity may allow for the generation of additional revenue as well.

Policy measures called for the imposition of taxes on foods of poor nutritional quality, such as carbonated soft drinks and high-fat foods. Countries where this is an important problem discussed the need for measures to regulate the sale of high-fat meat and meat products. There were also proposals for the creation of laws and regulations protecting consumers against the dangers of high levels of exposure to additives used in the production of processed foods, e.g. monosodium glutamate and borax; and against the unhygienic manufacture and processing of food products.

The need for policy restricting commercial food advertising to children was also pointed out, as well as the need to enable the public to judge the advertising put out by the beauty and fitness ventures.

Delegates representing vast populations entrenched in poverty addressed the need to adjust national food structures in order to be more equitably responsive to food supply needs and demands. They also called for laws protecting national food resources, while a proposal was made for the provision of incentives and subsidies improving access to healthy foods. A suggestion was also made to use food tax revenues for disease prevention.

Towards the improvement of health services, the majority of Member States seek (or propose) to reduce child mortality rates by giving due focus to new programmes designed to raise awareness among mothers, children and young people about health risks as a consequence of poor diet and physical inactivity, by promoting health during the early stages of life, i.e. intra-uterine, infancy, childhood and adolescence. Additional creative strategies suggested include periodic physical fitness tests within settings such as schools and written prescriptions for physical activity from general practitioners.

Representatives strongly supported such regional initiatives as the Jogyakarta Declaration for a Healthy ASEAN 2020 and the ASEAN Health Ministers' meeting in Vientiane, Lao People's Democratic Republic in March 2002. In the meetings in Jogyakarta and Vientiane, attention was also given to the need to support policy with funding and infrastructure to allow the lifestyle changes being promoted to take place.

Finally, there was extensive recognition of the need for continuing research, data-gathering and scientific analysis of the interrelationships between unhealthy diet and physical inactivity on the one hand, and the prevalence of chronic diseases on the other. There was discussion about the need to be careful when extrapolating data from developed countries to developing countries, as well as to the need for culture- and population-specific approaches, interventions and policies.

Special points addressed to the WHO include the unanimous call for a coherent global strategy in stemming the perils of obesity-related diseases and the need to put this among its priorities, as well as to assistance in addressing international treaty organizations such as the World Trade Organization (WTO) in using food importation regulations to protect public health in developing countries in particular, and within the Region in general.

BARRIERS AND ACTIONS NEEDED TO IMPROVE HEALTH STATUS THROUGH DIET AND PHYSICAL ACTIVITY*

1.1 ON POLICY

Barriers	*Action*
Availability/introduction of new foods, e.g. Western-type fast foods; importable agricultural, meat and dairy products; processed foods, etc. (10)	Impose taxes on foods of poor nutritional quality, e.g. carbonated sweetened beverages and high-fat foods (1) Measures to regulate the sale of high-fat content meat and meat products (2) Create laws and regulations protecting consumers: • against the dangers of high levels of exposure to additives used in the production of processed foods, e.g. monosodium glutamate, borax (1) • against the unhygienic manufacture and processing of food products (2)
Poverty/prohibitive food costs (4)	Adjust the national food structure so that food may be supplied to consumers in a more comprehensive way (3) Protect national food resources (2) Provide incentives and subsidies to improve access to healthy foods (1)

*Numbers in parenthesis indicate how many representatives mentioned each barrier and action.

Barriers	*Action*
Misconception that public health is the concern of health ministries alone (1)	Integrate health promotion into national policies involving health, agriculture, development, education, housing, town planning, sports, human resources, transport, tourism (8)
	Make health impact assessments an integral policy requirement for all major planning and development processes, e.g. a study on the impact on a community's eating choices and recreational space and activities brought about by new buildings, facilities, shopping centres, transport system, roads (5)
	Build strategic partnerships: • across all levels of government, industry and nongovernment sectors (10) • involving grocery organizations, school canteens, fast food outlets, etc to promote healthy lifestyles, particularly those affecting the eating behaviour of children and young people (6) • especially with the food industry, approach must be of that towards a partner and not as towards an adversary in promoting and facilitating healthy eating and lifestyles (5)

*Numbers in parenthesis indicate how many representatives mentioned each barrier and action.

1.2 ON AWARENESS-RAISING*

Barriers	*Actions*
Poor public awareness on nutrition (7) "Knowledge-behaviour" paradox (2) Traditions and customs (1)	Integrate health promotion initiatives into healthy settings, e.g. home, pre-school, school, and workplace (10) Develop creative and relevant communications strategies for increasing health promotion and public awareness on nutrition and physical activity (11) Provide incentives, e.g. awards and prizes, for excellent health promotion programmes and initiatives (3) Promote consumer education through food labeling and product information (8) Promote and popularize, through education, traditional healthy cooking techniques using healthy ingredients as alternative (5) Promote physical fitness campaigns using traditional dances and martial arts as popular vehicles (3)
Media, e.g. fast-food advertisements, commercials on cigarette smoking and alcohol consumption, on fashionable slimness among women, that "fat babies are beautiful" (8) Inadequate diets, especially among women and adolescents with poor body image (2)	Create laws and regulations restricting commercial food advertising to children (1) Promote health through role models, e.g. government officials, national personalities, sports celebrities, etc (5) Create laws and regulations protecting public health against the commercial exploitation by health, beauty and fitness markets (1)

*Numbers in parenthesis indicate how many representatives mentioned each barrier and action.

1.3 ON IMPROVING THE ENVIRONMENT *

Barriers	*Actions*
Lifestyle changes, e.g. from an agricultural setting to the office environment (7)	Invest in infrastructure development towards the creation of environments that enable and promote physical activities (6)
Change in dietary patterns, due mainly to the increase in employment rate among women (3)	Create laws and regulations against smoking in public areas (3)
Higher income and better standards of living (9)	Promote creatively organized national fitness events, e.g. walkathons, hiking aces, etc (8)
Technological advancement, e.g. the proliferation of motorized vehicles, lifts and labour-saving devices (9)	
Diminishing/insufficient infrastructure for recreational activities, e.g. parks, pedestrian areas, etc (6)	Form commercial partnerships that may lead to fund generation to augment the dwindling financial resources of health ministries and for the development of other public health facilities (3)
Poor hygiene and sanitation, lack of clean water (2)	Deduct income tax for expenses in physical fitness activities (1)

*Numbers in parenthesis indicate how many representatives mentioned each barrier and action.

1.4 ON IMPROVING HEALTH SERVICES *

Barriers	*Actions*
The "double-burden" of disease: continuing battle against communicable diseases alongside the emerging prevalence of noncommunicable diseases (NCDs) (4)	Position health promotion as a regional concern, e.g. the Jogyakarta Declaration in 2000 on healthy ASEAN 2020, the March 2002 ASEAN Health Ministers' Meeting in Vientiane, Lao People's Democratic Republic (4)
Asymptomatic nature of NCDs until the late stages of the diseases' progress (1)	Reduce child mortality rates by focusing on new programmes in awareness-raising for mothers, children and young people on health risks throughout life as consequences of poor diet and physical inactivity (i.e. a *life course emphasis*) by approaching health promotion through the early stages of life: intra-uterine, infancy, childhood, adolescence (10)
Improved diagnosis and management of diseases threaten to upset health budgets due to long and expensive treatment costs (4)	
	Conduct periodic physical fitness tests within settings, e.g. schools, workplaces, etc (1)
	Promote physical fitness among people with sedentary lifestyles and NCDs through written prescriptions from general practitioners (1)
	Create a disease prevention fund from food tax revenues (1)

*Numbers in parenthesis indicate how many representatives mentioned each barrier and action.

Barriers	*Actions*
Inadequate support for nutrition research (1) Lack of trained health professionals in nutrition and physical activity (1)	Position health promotion as a national policy agenda; support policy with funding and infrastructure (11) Promote and continue the conduct of research and data-gathering on the interrelationships of unhealthy diet, physical inactivity and NCDs along national, regional and international levels, including baseline data-gathering at national and sub-national levels (7) Create culture- and population-specific approaches, interventions and policies (1) Caution against extrapolating data from developed countries to developing countries (1)

Summary of other comments:*

Poor nutrition/diet and physical inactivity cause:

- Obesity-related diseases such as cardiovascular diseases, diabetes mellitus, and cancer (18)

- Risks to reproductive health and low-birth-weight babies, especially when combined with smoking (4)

- Risks to health throughout life (8)

*Numbers in parenthesis indicate how many representatives mentioned each barrier and action.

Recommendations to WHO*:

- Develop a coherent global strategy in combating chronic diseases and make this a priority (18)

- Continue strengthening the ASEAN-WHO collaboration in resource mobilization and technical support (4)

- Provide technical assistance at both country and regional levels on health promotion focusing on the prevention of NCDs

  - provide assistance in strengthening a national health promotion programme (2)

  - facilitate exchange of best practices and positive experiences among countries (2)

  - provide technical support and assistance in the prevention and control of NCDs, specifically regarding epidemiological information on NCDs (1)

  - assist in establishing national and sub-national data on the prevalence of NCDs (1)

- Focus health promotion efforts on the need for proper diet and physical activity particularly on the early stages of life, i.e. intra-uterine, infancy and childhood (3)

- Assist in empowering health ministries in revenue generation (2)

- Assist in addressing international trade treaty organizations, e.g. the World Trade Organization, against the importation of high fat-content foodstuff by developing countries, e.g. mutton flaps, turkey tails and other fatty meats (1)

*Numbers in parenthesis indicate how many representatives mentioned each barrier and action.